FROM THE DESK OF MS. ODESS

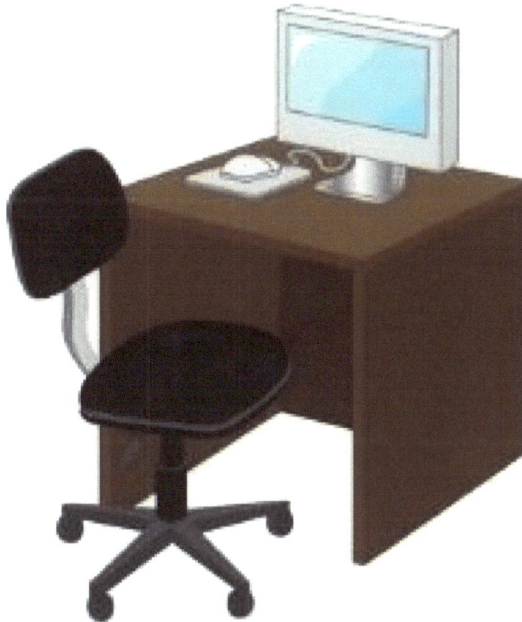

HEALTH AND WELLNESS BELONGS TO US ALL

ALL THE NATURAL HERBS, SPICES, OILS AND FRAGRANCE THAT WERE USED FROM THE BEGINNING OF TIME

Odessa frankson

INTRODUCTION

Ms. Odessa Frankson RN/Nurse Practioner:
Administrator of: Wisdom Home Care Agency.
BSN. MSN. HONORARY MASTERS AND PHD.

We subscribe to the concept of health organization which is "not merely the absence of disease or infirmity but a state of complete physical, mental, and social wellbeing.

Mission Statement: We believe, the enjoyment of the highest attainable standard of health is one of the fundamental rights of every human being without distinction of race, color, religion, sexual orientation, national origin, physical or mental handicap, marital status, military or political affiliation and economic or social condition.

I believe a person's health is important. I've learned a lot about natural elements and herbs that have proven to be beneficial in many ways. I want to share this with everyone, so I decided that I would write about the different natural remedies and their benefits. I have tried and experienced the benefits of most of these natural remedies.

I'm not taking away from medication that has been described to anyone. I believe that healing comes from (some) medication; eating right and taking care of yourself.

HERBS TO FLUSH OUT BODY POISONS

HERBS

We can recharge our winter-weary mind and body, and melt away unwanted pounds with cleansing herbal remedies that will make us as frisky as we should be.

To revive a tired body, we should give ourselves a refreshed appearance in order to have youthful energy; we should try some of these herbal boosters.

Stimulates

>ECHINACEA: This herb stimulates the sweat glands to purify the blood and helps boost the body's immune system to respond quickly to illness and infection.

>LICORICE ROOT: A blood purifier, body organ cleanser, and liver stimulant, licorice root contains a substance which curbs cravings for sweets and helps control the appetite as well.

>SARSAPARILLA: Another sweat gland stimulant that helps to cleanse the body of poisons and is also rich in vital plant hormones.

>FENNEL: Mild fennel soothes stomach distress, especially the uncomfortable feeling sometimes caused by dieting. It helps flush out excess water from the tissues and speeds up the body's ability to expel impurities during dieting

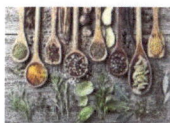

>CHICKWEED: Washes out accumulations of lactic acid, helps revive and pep up tired muscles and is a superior appetite suppressant which helps dieters avoid hunger pangs.

>ALOE VERA: Well known as a healing plant, it soothes the liver, stomach, kidney and bladder, and makes a superior skin ointment valuable for sunburn, burned skin rashes, irritations and minor cuts and bruises.

>BURDOCK ROOT: Considered the king of body purifier's burdock root helps flush out toxic wastes and accumulated body poisons and makes you feel young and full of zip.

>CAPSICUM: Stimulates circulation, helps loosen mucus and cholesterol and dissolves fatty deposits, Capsicum also helps strengthen blood vessels and creates an overall feeling of rejuvenation.

>DANDELION ROOT: This root can be grounded up and used as a caffeine-free coffee substitute. Many Herbalists say it cleanses vital body organs, flushes out excess fluids, cleanses the blood and makes a highly effective rejuvenating tonic.

>FENUGREEK: This herb taste like celery; it helps soothe inflammations of the gastrointestinal system, and it lubricates the lining of the intestines and assists in the

elimination of mucus. A teaspoon in a cup of warm water makes an excellent gargle for sore throats.

REFRESHES

Refreshers

>GOLEN SEAL: This herb stimulates sluggish muscles, soothes digestive problems and clears up respiratory congestion. By cleansing the lungs and nasal passages it refreshes the body and the mind.

>GINSENG: Rejuvenates glands and enhances our production of vital hormones, peps-up sluggish body functions, and provides an overall youthful feeling.

>BLADDERWRACK: Removes obstructions and washes them out of the system. It's especially valuable to dieters because it regulates the thyroid, a key to weight control.

>BUCHU LEAF: Contains unique oil, a powerful cleanser and flusher of fat and body poisons. It promotes clear thinking and it rejuvenates the system by its cleansing action.

>CHAMOMILE: Often used as a natural painkiller, it also has [antispasmatic] qualities which helps soothe hunger pangs during dieting, and it also helps flush fat from the body.

VITALITY

VITALITY

>YARROW: An internal astringent which detoxifies the system, helps soothe respiratory problems, opens the pores, and rids the body of accumulated waste. It has also been used to cleanse the body's vital organs. It promotes an overall feeling of youth and vitality.

"Herbs are becoming a more and more important factor in today's health care," I heard a Doctor say, and I totally agree.

Enjoy a body that is free of pollution and fat with the help of these plant foods.

These potent herbal healers can be used as teas, syrups, or powders to sprinkle over food.

ODD SYMPTOMS!

ODD SYMPTONS!

RESTLESS LEGS: Try iron, this is the most common nutrient shortfall in women. It can make nerves in the legs super sensitive causing restless, squirmy sensation. Taking 18mg to 25mg daily can stop the squirminess in about 90 days.

WEAK HANDS: Try vitamin B-12. A daily dose 1,000 mcg can relieve carpal tunnel syndrome, weakness, and numbness up to 80%. This vitamin helps your nerves function at its peak.

<u>CHILLY & SLUGGISH</u>: Your system may be low on iodine. It helps to keep your body energized and warm. Adding 100 mcg iodine supplement daily or adding ½ tsp. of iodized salt to your daily diet can correct a shortfall, ending tiredness and chills within 3 months

<u>MUSCLE CRAMPS:</u> Try magnesium, it helps muscles contract and relax properly when you're in motion. Muscle tics, cramps, charley horses, if our legs are dip! Take 40mg of magnesium supplement daily.

AMAZING BIBLE OIL CURE FOR ARTHRITIS

AMAZING BIBLE OIL CURE FOR ARTHRITIS
(The Bible tells us that people in ancient times regarded frankincense very highly)

A New miracle capsule with an ancient ingredient treasured in the days of Jesus Christ turns out to be a godsend for arthritis.

It's a form of Frankincense, the oil that the Magi laid at the feet of Jesus.

Amazed modern researchers say that it ends the agony of arthritis quickly by shrinking inflamed tissue.

The breakthrough medication is called Boswellia, a type of frankincense oil taken from India's Boswellia Tree.

In one study at the Government Medical College in Jammu India, a whopping 70 percent of arthritis patients tested had a dramatic turn around.

Three quarters of them had been bedridden, but within a few weeks they were able to get out of bed and grip things that before would have triggered excruciating pain.

In another study of 26 patients with arthritis knee joints, a major improvement was reported after four weeks.

Boswellia is taking America by storm. Dr. E.W. McDougal of Kansas City gave it to 350 pain-wracked patients

People taking multiple kinds of medication developed side effects, from them; but, once they started taking Boswellia, pain was significantly reduced, or even completely gone in two to four weeks. All patients were able to drop other medication or reduce the dosage of the medication they were taking.

It has been reported that a 56 year old woman who tried varies medications, had no known results. Then she began taking the Boswellia capsules and they brought her the relief she needed. Boswellia has no side effects.
That's a wonderful blessing! Other arthritis drugs can irritate blood pressure, heart rate or messes with your stomach. Bosweilla doesn't cost a fortune.
You can get it from your health food store.

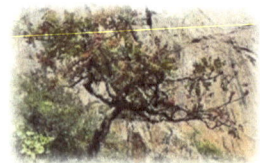

Energizing fragrances

Fragrances from herbs, spices flowers can help you prevent tiredness and fatigue forever!

The symptoms of Chronic Fatigue syndrome (CFS) includes: tiredness, weakness, muscular pain, fevers, chills, depression, mood swings, stresses and sleep disturbance.

Aromatherapy: healing through inhaling certain odors, is elegant, pleasurable and one of the most consistently successful ways to relieve the symptoms of CFS.

The simplicity of aromatherapy (it is its greatest virtue). You can dab these pure oils inside your nostrils, place a drop on a radiator, candle or light bulb, add them to your basic massage oil; or, scent your bath water with a few drops. There are dozens of natural oils, each with a different therapeutic value, and you can combine them to develop many new scents. Stick to using single oils until you've found the ones that work for you; then combine them in equal proportions. Use these natural oils to banish tiredness and stress from your life; they can be found in most health food stores.

>LAVENDER: This light and flowery fragrance soothes the mind and body. A few drops in the bath helps you sleep.

>LEMON: A fresh cool fragrance that calms the mind and helps prevent fevers.

>LEMON-LAVENDER Mix: Works like knockout drops to produce undisturbed sleep.

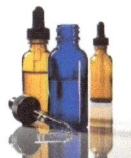

>PEPPERMINT: This invigorating scent energizes mind and body and helps digestion.

>Basil: Another energizer; it lifts the spirit and clears the mind.

ROSEMARY: A sniff of this herb can improve your memory, and it's a clean, sharp fragrance that relieves lethargy and early-morning sluggishness.

>CLARY SAGE: This nutty, floral scent soothes and lifts the spirit.

>ORANGE/SWEET ORANGE: A refreshing fragrance, that helps you to feel stronger mentally and physically.

>GERANIUM/ROSE GERANIUM: Soothing floral scents that cleanses both mind and body and eases troubled emotions.

"If you plan to apply basil or peppermint oils in your shin, as in a massage, they should be diluted beforehand," but, all of these oils, can be diluted with vegetable oil without losing their therapeutic effect.

"For the ultimate in luxurious skin care, you should dilute the essences with oil of sweet almond or almond oil."

Only tiny quantities of oil exist in each plant, so hundreds of plants must be processed to produce a bottle of fatigue killing pure essence.

Nothing (yet known) permanently alleviates CFS, and until we find something that does, the relief provided by aromatherapy will allow you to think and feel positive; a major factor in your favor on a day to day basis. But none of the oils should be taken internally, except under medical supervision.

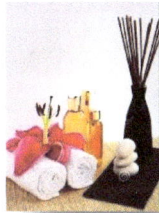

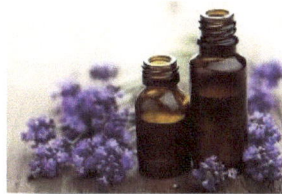

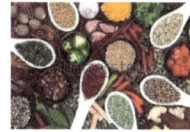

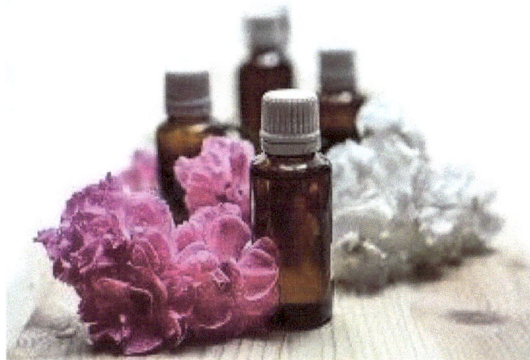

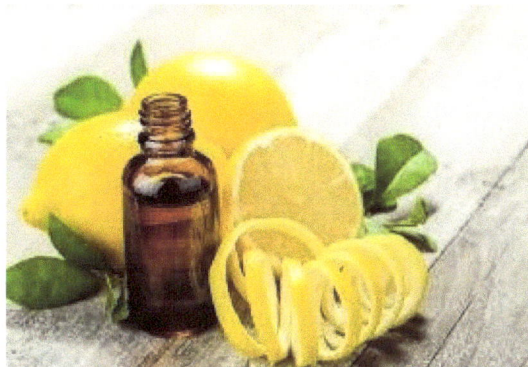

KELP THE HEALTH GIVER

(Life on this planet had its genesis in the waters. Genesis 1:20 says, "And God said, let the waters bring forth……..")

It seems logical to assume that life began in the waters and the seas; which contain vital agents that promote biological activities that produce benefits in multiple areas.

"The science of biochemistry proves that all life, and of all life forms thrown up by the seas the common seaweed known as Kelp deserves special attention."

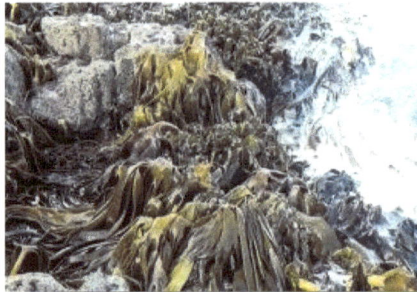

Common names:
Bladder wrack, Seaweed, Kelp
Bladder Fucus, Kelware.
Botanical description:
Fucus Vesiculosus

KELP AS A MEDICINE

Kelp has been employed in medicine for a very long time by both the orthodox and the herbal schools.

Fucus Vesiculosus contains about 0.1 percent of volatile oil, cellulose, mucilage, mannite, colouring and bitter principles, sodium and potassium.

These saline ingredients constitute 14 to 20 percent of ashes. It has also been stated that a small quantity of a sugar named Focuses exists in the dried Kelp.

Fucus acts on obesity mainly through the thyroid, which gland it tends to normalize. Thyroid trouble can cause obesity and it can also cause excessive thinness.

Not only does Fucus act on the thyroid, but it most certainly has a remedial and normalizing action on the sensory nerves, meninges, arteries, pylorus, colon, liver, gall bladder, pancreas, bile duct, kidneys, prostate gland, uterus, fat cells, testicles and ovaries. Fucus can be taken causing no harm or side effects. However Fucus also known as Kelp, works better when taken in small doses, especially if any of the organs mentioned happen to be "diseased."

Suggested dosage: 1x or 2x (potency in tablet form two or three times a day).

KELP AND THE TISSUE SALTS

KELP AND THE TISSUE SALTS

Fucus has an even better action in many instances and for general tonic purposes when it is blended with the tissue salts of Schuessler. The plant acts as a sort of vehicle for the cell salt; and the results are satisfactory.

A person suffering from calcium deficiency the use of calcium rich foods and the tissue salt Calcium Phosphate produced no results; but when Kelp was taken with the salt, assimilation took place.

KELP IN NERVOUS DISORDER

KELP IN NERVOUS DISORDER

There is no doubt that some nervous complaints are due to a deficiency of certain cell salts, especially those of phosphorus, potassium, iron, sodium and the elements of lead, copper, silver and zinc. In other words, many nervous troubles are "deficiency diseases" and should respond to correct nutrition and a diet rich in the essential nerve building minerals.

The nerve cases where Kelp was helpful are too numerous to mention. A bad case of neurasthenia was reported, where a 24 year old was utterly exhausted. The young man had nervous dyspepsia with much flatulence; he complained of pain in his back; he was constipated and could not sleep except in fitful snatches. Kelp played a vital part in his total recovery. Of course he was placed on a suitable diet, given gentle breathing and other exercises supported with psychological aid: but there was no real change in his condition until he took kelp with his meals three times daily. He also took cell salts of Kali Phos., Natrum Phos., Natrum Mur., and Silica.

KELP IN HEADACHES

KELP IN HEADACHES

A lady who was having headaches was tested (by means of Radiesthesia); it revealed trouble of meninges: inflammation of the meninges which never developed. The doctor's medication cured the trouble in the early stages. After using Rediesthesia it was found that Kelp was the remedy. The dosage of Kelp was given in homeopathic potency for two weeks and the pain vanished. Studies show that many cases involving the skull have responded to Kelp treatment. Kelp has helped in many cases of migraine pain, but as other remedies were employed, Kelp only played a part in removing the cause of the trouble.

KELP IN ARTERIAL TROUBLES & HIGH BLOOD PRESSURE

Kelp is an arterial cleansing agent that gives tone to the walls of the blood vessels. It is helpful in some cases of arterial tension (high blood pressure).

Some Practitioners believe that it helps to remove deposits from the walls of the arteries and restores its elasticity, thereby lengthening life.

It normalizes low blood pressure.

INDIGESTION AND THE PYLORUS

INDIGESTION AND THE PYLORUS

Where there is contraction (spasm) or congestion in the pylorus (small intestine), nutrients can't pass as freely as they should from the stomach to the next stage: digestion/assimilation. Kelp is a most useful remedy for almost all troubles with pylorus. I repeat that for this purpose: small doses act better than large quantities; indeed the small dose is superior in almost all instances and the pulverized herb is better than extract.

KELP FOR WEAKNESS OF THE COLON

KELP FOR WEAKNESS OF THE COLON

A host of physical disorders and even some forms of insanity are due to toxemia coming from a foul colon. Poisons accumulate in this large bowel and absorbs into the blood stream causing debility, rheumatism, nervous disorders; kidney trouble and all those complaints due to disorganized, toxic blood.

Reformed healers pay much attention to cleansing the colon with enemas and high colonic irrigation, and a great deal of good has been accomplished by such methods. However, these cleansing processes do not contribute very much to toning up the colon so that it can get rid of its accumulated poisons unaided. A toxic colon is a weak colon and needs to be built up.

There are many remedies that perform this service, but certainly not purgatives, which only weaken the organ (still further). Among a number of very excellent colonic agents Kelp must take its place with the best. The reason why this sea plant has a toning action is probably due to its high natural mineral salt content. The salts build the walls of the organ and the iodine. For this reason, Kelp is advised in all cases and diseases associated with auto-toxemia (self-poisoning). All constipated people should take Kelp daily, and its action should be assisted Black Molasses.

KELP VITALIZES THE IMPORTANT ORGANS

THE LIVER

The Liver is very sensitive to mental states; the mind also reacts to the liver. To be bright and vital, one must have an active liver. This organ is very important to normal health; much constipation (which is the cause of auto-toxemia) is due to liver troubles.

Kelp is an "organ remedy" for the liver. That is to say it has an affinity for the organ and has a direct action upon it. The action of this remedy is to supply the liver with the salts it needs for normal function, and it also has a sweetening and cleansing affect.

Note: Kelp acts on the liver and colon; hence its value is obvious to all who are costive, toxic, depressed and "out of sorts."

It has been known that many very obstinate liver conditions yield to the influence of Kelp, but the sufferer must eat sensibly if any good results are to be maintained.

GALL BLADDER

GALL BLADDER

As a rule anything which helps the liver, aids the gall bladder, but not always. However, Kelp acts on both organs and has proved to be very effective in clearing an obstructed gall bladder. It is probable that the highly evolved sodium content of the remedy plays a large part in this connection. I cannot totally say that Kelp has any value in cases of gall stones as I have never tried it on its own. But it seems reasonable to suppose that any remedy which tones the liver and gall bladder will have some good effects in these cases and will at least help to prevent the formation of stones.

THE PANCREAS

THE PANCREAS

Many people who suffer from indigestion and constitutional weakness may have a weak pancreas.

Kelp, taken regularly, will help to keep the pancreas in order and may well prevent more serious organic diseases from developing later on.

Very often, in my professional work cases where (although) there is no sugar in the urine, the pancreas functions poorly; Kelp is one of the best organ remedies for a sluggish pancreas.

A group of people who practice Radiesthesia, placed Kelp high on their list of remedies for pancreatic troubles; its constant use can't do any harm irrespective of age or condition.

THE BILE DUCT

THE BILE DUCT

We cannot leave our discussion (of the action of Kelp on the digestive organs) without giving brief mention of its value as a remedy for obstruction of the bile duct. But as this is of little interest to the layman it will serve if I merely state that the action of this remedy is profound and that it has done excellent work in this connection to my certain knowledge.

THE KIDNEYS

THE KIDNEYS

The ancients paid more attention to the health of the kidneys than we do today.

Of recent years we have found that the kidneys are not only eliminative organs; they also aid in assimilation and are partly responsible for adequate nutrition.

Also, it must be remembered that the vital suprarenal glands are situated on the top of the kidneys. These glands secrete adrenalin and play a large part in supplying us with vitality, and meet the demands for extra energy at times of stress and exertion. Anything which helps to keep the kidneys healthy must (we assume) also aid the suprarenal.

Kelp certainly cleanses and tones; these organs are especially valuable when the kidneys are in an "irritable" state and painful. Kelp has helped to clear up a lot of kidney cases that were very stubborn, and that had failed to respond to other treatments; naturopathic herbal and biochemical.

PROSTATE GLAND

Kelp for prostate gland trouble, that's surely a new idea! This remedy will do much to normalize a weak and enlarged prostate gland. To the experienced biochemist the chemical composition of the remedy explains (just) why.

Many men faced with operations for prostate trouble could be spared this ordeal if they took Kelp regularly, especially after the age of forty.

The action of Kelp on the prostate is to improve the nutrition of the organ and the circulation of the blood through the tissues. "The blood is the life" and in common with all other organs, the health of the prostate depends on the normal circulation of chemically balanced blood through its substance.

The value of Kelp in this connection has been proved by the excellent results obtained; but it is necessary to take the food remedy over time, and wise to keep it up.

THE UTERUS

THE UTERUS

The organ which develops into the prostate gland in the male becomes the uterus in the female.

It is natural that we find Kelp to be a most useful agent for toning up a weak uterus. Of the ten vegetable remedies that employs for weakness of this organ, Kelp is most valuable (especially) when the sufferer is troubled with associated nervous disorders and depression.

In some medical opinions, Kelp would be of value to pregnant women, and help promote normal deliveries.

THE TESTICLES

THE TESTICLES

We find Kelp again performing a service not formerly thought of: hardening of the testes and simple impotency; this remedy should produce good results if taken consistently. It does not over stimulate and it cannot harm. No doubt the value lies in the improved local circulation of blood rich in cell salts.

In cases of impotent men, Kelp treatment was given with varying degrees of satisfaction; but, it must be remembered that the causes of impotency are complex and often include the psychological side; too much shouldn't be expected of Kelp or any other remedy in the treatment of this type of trouble.

THE OVARIES

Kelp accomplishes the same results for the ovaries as it does for weakness of the uterus. More often than not, the two troubles go together and what aids one organ directly affects the others.

For ovarian pain, irregular menses, depression, and even in some cases of anemia, Kelp is found most helpful. The food remedy should be taken for several weeks or months; the normalizing process (although slow) is in harmony with natural law and usually produces reason to believe that the constant use of Kelp may prevent growths and ovarian cysts; but, it is not held out as a cure for such conditions.

The use of Kelp for female depression alone is well worth a thorough trial.

KELP AND THE THYROID

KELP AND THE THYROID

Kelp has been known for the need of iodine, in the treatment of thyroid gland trouble.

The Greeks ate sponges and other sea plants to cure goiter, but it was not until 1849 that Chatin established a connection between iodine deficiency and goiter.

Later, iodine was discovered in the thyroid, and it was detertmined that in people suffering from goiter there was an iodine deficiency.

With the exception of sea foods, most articles of diet are lacking in iodine. Fish oils contain iodine, but Kelp is probably the best source. Too much iodine may produce over-activity of the thyroid, which leads to mental excitement and emotionalism; this is one reason why you only advocate small doses of iodine products.

KELP FOR COUGHS, COLDS AND WEAK LUNGS

KELP FOR COUGHS, COLDS AND WEAK LUNGS
It has been said that certain herbal remedies can make short work of this troublesome malady by promoting elimination through perspiration. Also the Homeopaths and Naturopaths can hasten cure of the acute condition and help to prevent colds by building up vitality, generally.

As with other ailments: those who suffer from continual colds, coughs and catarrh, are suffering from a cell salt deficiency, and they also lack sufficient iodine. I'm not holding out Kelp as a cure for the acute cough and cold, but, the constant use of Kelp is very likely to increase the resistance of these maladies that the system will in due course become free of.

THE BEST WAY IN WHICH TO TAKE KELP

Long experience has proven that most herbal remedies have a much deeper action when they are potentised homeopathically. By this process the real healing power of the remedy is "liberated," and a tiny dose produces far better effects than the larger doses of the same item in crude form. Crude and potentised preparations have been used for many years and I am convinced that the potentised article has a much deeper and prolonged action on the system. This is true of Kelp in potency. In some cases where the crude article gave but little aid, the employment of the 1x potency produced satisfactory results, especially when combined with indicated potentised mineral salts.

The system can deal with and take up a remedy in potentised form when it fails to react to the crude material dose.

CONCLUSION ABOUT KELP

CONCLUSION ABOUT KELP

"This plant has a reputation as an artifact, claiming that it diminishes the fat without injuring the health. It influences the mucus membranes and the lymphatics. It is a gently stimulating and toning alterant. It is one of those slow, persistent agents that require time to accomplish the desired result.

It is stimulating to the absorbents and especially influences the fatty globules. Its best action is observed in individuals having a cold, torpid, clammy skin and loose flabby rolls of fat. It is an agent that gives better results in cases of morbid obesity than in those cases of healthy character. It is best to begin with small doses.

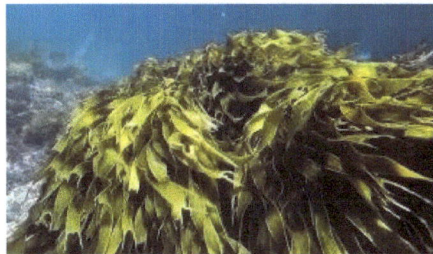

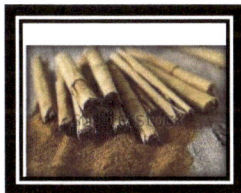

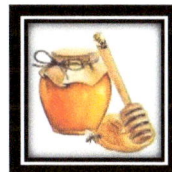

CINNAMON AND HONEY

CINNAMON AND HONEY

The combination of honey and cinnamon has been used for centuries in both traditional Chinese and Ayurveda, a system of healing found thousands of years ago in India.

(These two ingredients with unique healing abilities have a long history as a home remedy.) Cinnamon has been known as one of the oldest spices to mankind, and honey's popularity has continued throughout history.

Cinnamon's essential oils and honey's enzyme that produces hydrogen peroxide qualify the two "anti-microbial" foods with the ability to help stop the growth of bacteria as well as fungi.

Both are used not just as a beverage flavoring and medicine, but also as an embalming agent and it is used as alternatives to traditional food preservatives due to their effective antimicrobial properties.

Also, it is worth mentioning that in Ayurveda medicine, honey known as 'Yogavahi', which means "the carrier of the healing values of the herbs to our cells and tissues". It is believed that when combined with another substance (e.g. herb or spice) in a formulation, the special quality of honey enhances the medicinal qualities of that formulation and it helps them reach the deeper tissues in the body more effectively.

Honey and cinnamon, which is one of the best-known mixtures, has been reported to be a natural cure for many diseases and formula for many health benefits.

ARTHRITIS: Apply a paste made of the two ingredients on the affected part of the body and massage slowly.

Drinking tea with honey and cinnamon daily can also help relieve pain and stiffness in the joints.

HEART DISEASES: Apply honey and cinnamon powder, on bread instead of using jam or butter and eat it regularly for breakfast. It is believed that in the long run, this can help prevent blockages in blood vessels, heart attacks and hypercholesterolemia.

HAIR LOSS: Apply a paste of hot olive oil, a tablespoon of honey, a teaspoon of cinnamon powder before bath; leave it for 15 min and wash.

BLADDER INFECTIONS: Mix a teaspoon of cinnamon powder and half a teaspoon of honey in a glass of lukewarm water and drink. This can help destroy the bacteria in the urinary system.

TOOTHACHE: Apply a paste of cinnamon powder and honey on the aching tooth.

CHOLESTEROL: Add honey to cinnamon powder mixed in boiled water or green tea, and drink.

COLDS: Make a glass of lukewarm honey water mixed with a pinch of cinnamon powder to help boost your immune system during the cold season. It is also helpful in clearing the sinuses.

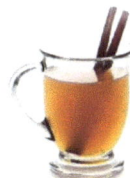

INDIGESTION: Cinnamon powder sprinkled on a spoonful of honey taken before food, relieves acidity and prevents indigestion.

LONGEVITY: Regularly drink tea with honey and a little cinnamon powder to strengthen your immune system and protect your body from viral and bacterial attacks.

PIMPLES: Mix honey with cinnamon powder; apply the paste on the pimples before sleeping; wash away, the next morning.

OBESITY: To reduce weight: drink daily a teaspoon of honey with half a teaspoon of cinnamon powder boiled in water; drink it on an empty stomach in the morning (about half an hour before breakfast).
Step-by-step instructions: CINNAMON AND HONEY RECIPE.

Cinnamon has an insulin boosting property (water soluble compounds called polyphenol type A polymers) which has the ability to boost insulin activity about 20 fold and can benefit people who have high sugar levels (obese people, pre-diabetics and diabetics).

Also, read the Honey Hibernation Diet Theory to find out how honey contributes to the metabolizing of undesirable cholesterol and fatty acid. It provides a fueling mechanism for the body, and keeps blood sugar levels balanced; and it allows recovery hormones to burn stored body fat.

BAD BREATH: Gargle with honey and cinnamon powder mixed in warm water so that breath stays fresh throughout the day.

Honey plus cinnamon together; besides being an amazing potential cure for so many illnesses, their total fragrant sweet and warm taste is a perfect match for the palate. The combination adds a magic effect to the taste of cakes, breads, biscuits and rolls; and is known to make many winning recipes in the world of delicious foods, such as the famous, easy-to-make, kids' favorite classic - honey and cinnamon butter toast!

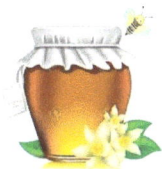

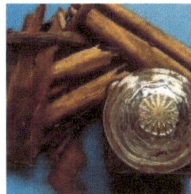

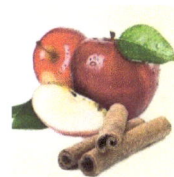

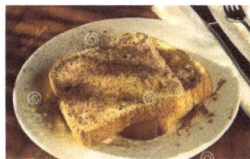

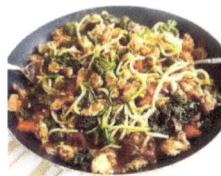

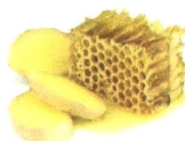

Some of the health benefits from Honey and Ginger Spice

ASTHMA: It is also believed that a mixture of honey and ginger, along with black pepper, is capable of treating or reducing the effects of asthma.

It is a naturally soothing and anti-inflammatory mix that releases the tension and promotes the flow of oxygen to the lungs and the relaxation of the blood vessels in the lungs.

RESPIRATORY PROBLEMS: The mixture of honey and ginger is an excellent expectorant and therefore provides instant relief to people suffering from cough, cold, sore throat, and runny nose.

CANCER MANAGEMENT:
Ginger has been linked recently to a reduction in nausea and vomiting that is associated with cancer and chemotherapy treatments.

Patients often suffer debilitating nausea following these intense procedures, and they often turn to alternative solutions to eliminate it. Ginger speeds up the emptying of the stomach through its digestive properties, which can prevent the discomfort and probability of nausea.

Nausea from chemotherapy is caused by cisplatin, a primary chemotherapy component; ginger can balance out its powerful effect. Ginger has also been positively connected with reducing the nausea and vomiting that is associated with "**pregnancy**" and "morning sickness." This, combined with the naturally soothing effects of honey, makes for a powerful preventative solution to vomiting and nausea caused from various sources.

CANCER PREVENTION: In terms of cancer prevention, studies have shown that the combination of honey and ginger result in **chemo-preventive properties** and the stimulus of antioxidant enzymes that reduces the chance of cancer growth and metastasis. Therefore, a honey ginger tonic, not only helps to reduce the symptoms of chemotherapy, but also reduces the chance of getting cancer (and needing the treatments in the first place).

INDIGESTION: Ginger and honey are also available in the form of: ginger honey tonic. It is believed that this tonic (or syrup) is a good digestive aid due to the inherent digestive **properties** of ginger. Furthermore, both ginger and honey have antioxidant properties; thereby increasing the strength of the body's immune system. Therefore, the consumption of one teaspoon of ginger and honey tonic is very useful for people who have a weak digestive system.

Ginger honey tonic has high levels of protein, which seriously **aids** in the digestive process; and it also stimulates the secretion of bile, which helps to dissolve fat. Furthermore, it stimulates the growth of intestinal flora, which speeds up the digestive process and facilitates proper bowel movements. Lastly, this gives a honey ginger tonic the ability to increase the absorption of other nutrients from **food** and reduces waste. For children, this has been **traditionally** given to ease stomach irritation because it is a very soothing solution, rather than traditional medicine.

<u>HEART HEALTH</u>:

The antioxidant properties of honey and ginger tonic have been shown to moderate prostaglandin behavior in the body. Prostaglandins are lipid compounds that are derived enzymatically from fatty acids, which are present in ginger. These prostaglandins are found throughout the body, and are functional elements in almost all organ systems. In terms of **heart** health, the moderating effects of honey and ginger tonic have shown a propensity to ease blood vessel tension, thereby reducing blood pressure and reducing the chance of conditions like atherosclerosis, heart attacks, and strokes.

For these reasons (and many more), people all around the world, especially in **India,** always keep both ginger and honey in their houses; they prepare this beneficial mixture when someone falls ill (with a cold or cough).

The best way to consume ginger and honey is to mix one teaspoon of ginger root juice with one teaspoon of honey.

Ginger honey crystals can also be purchased in markets and grocery stores. The crystallized ginger and honey that is pre-made, retains most of the health benefits presented in a fresh preparation and are meant for a quick and easy preparation of a ginger and honey beverage.

Ginger honey candies are also very popular. If your throat is congested and you are not able to speak properly, you should eat candied ginger and honey as it normally clears the throat immediately. Ginger honey candies are also useful during traveling, because they are known to help in dealing with motion sickness.

Honey can also be added to ginger to improve its taste. Honey acts as a sweetener, which makes ginger more palatable.

Honey can also be added to ginger bread, ginger cookies, ginger ale, ginger beer, carrot ginger soup, ginger punch, ginger biscuits, ginger snaps, ginger cake, and various other ginger recipes to enhance the taste of these recipes.

Honey is also often added to ginger root tea or ginger and cinnamon tea. You can replace sugar (if you're a sugar user) with honey, while preparing the ginger tea, thereby giving your ginger tea an extra healthy boost!

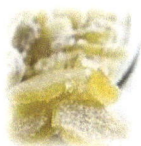

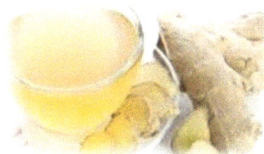

TURMERIC AND ITS BENEFITS

TURMERIC AND ITS BENEFITS

Studies show that turmeric curcumin can help *promote healthy joints, keep our hearts in top shape, and maintain* our cognitive functioning. Researchers are also suggesting that, when taken as a supplement, it can help keep our *immune system* balanced and working correctly.

TURMERIC CURCUMIN AND WHAT IT IS ALL ABOUT

TURMERIC CURCIMIN AND WHAT IT IS ALL ABOUT

For thousands of years, turmeric curcumin has been used in many ways over many millennia. First originating as a dye, and then repurposed as a medicinal component, turmeric curcumin has been a trusted and respected:

Health-Supporting Supplement for many years (and counting). Turmeric is well loved in medical circles for its healthful abilities to support and defend joint, bone, and physical wellness.

As a concentrated extract, turmeric curcumin contains antioxidant properties that help the body fight against free radicals, while possessing a far-reaching capacity to enhance full-body health.

Turmeric has been known to promote healthy functioning cognitive ability, enhance mood, empower whole body mobility and flexibility, as well as provide heart-related cardiovascular benefits. Turmeric curcumin supports the immune system, helps stabilize blood sugar, and even assists digestive function.

TURMERIC CURCUMIN POSSESSES ABILITIES:

1. It will, Support Joint and Bone health
2. Enhance cognitive functioning
3. Give the Benefit of Cardiovascular health
4. Bolster immune system defenses
5. It can Fight free radicals within our bodies
6. It will Promote Mobility and Flexibility
7. It Helps regulate the Digestive System
8. It provides Antioxidant health benefits
9. Optimize comfort in the Hands and Feet
10. It will Empower Positive overall well-being

All of the great health benefits are worth giving Turmeric a try!

WHAT WE NEED IN A TURMERIC CURCUMIN SUPPLEMENT

WHAT WE NEED IN A TURMERIC CURCUMIN SUPPLEMENT
Taking the *healthful attributes* listed above into consideration, here's a list of six characteristics we should look for in a great turmeric curcumin supplement. Try to seek out all of these qualities:

1. POWERFUL AND POTENCY

1000 mg of pure turmeric curcumin per day is the <u>minimum recommended daily serving size</u> that has been evidenced by numerous clinical studies to actually help your body thrive, even if you have to divide up the servings.

2. DOCTOR FORMULATED.

During our research of hundreds of products, we found that the highest quality, most effective turmeric curcumin supplements were all formulated by a respected doctor specializing in both nutrition and mobility.

3. MAXIMUM ABSORPTION

Curcumin is not an easy supplement for your body to absorb. <u>If you are not achieving maximum absorption, you might pass too much of it out of your system for it to be effective</u>. Bio-Perinea has been proven to assist absorption.

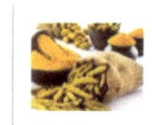

4. NO BINDERS OR FILLERS

Always ensure that the turmeric curcumin extract is plant-derived from a wholesome source, and that the top ingredient on the label is <u>pure turmeric curcumin</u>.

Binders, fillers, and additives are prevalent in cheap supplements and can be <u>unhealthy to ingest</u> and may counteract any desired outcome.

5. VEGETABLE CAPSULES

A truly wholesome turmeric curcumin supplement will be encapsulated in vegetarians—and, if possible; non-GMO plant-derived veggie capsules to guarantee an <u>effective, easy</u> and <u>safe</u>, delivery system, to your digestive tract.

6. NATURAL INGREDIENTS

It goes without saying; we want natural, pure, healthy ingredients in turmeric supplements that are backed by <u>pure, unadulterated turmeric curcumin extract</u>, so we know that we're getting the most authentic purity possible. All Natural ingredients are essential in any high-quality turmeric supplement.

THINGS TO AVOID WHEN TAKING TURMERIC

---

2 THINGS WE SHOULD AVOID WHEN TAKING TURMERIC

2 THINGS WE SHOULD AVOID WHEN TAKING TURMERIC

➤ GELATIN CAPSULES

These capsules are known to cause allergic reaction in many users. Worse, they're formulated from cows that may have been exposed to pesticides and antibiotics. Instead, try to find a turmeric curcumin formulated with vegetable capsules.

➢ FILLERS

Too many health brands have been cutting costs by using cheap additives that are harmful in their turmeric curcumin supplements. The top ones are: glycerin, caramel, and assorted oils.

We should also maintain a healthy eating lifestyle.

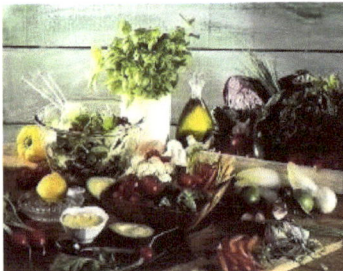

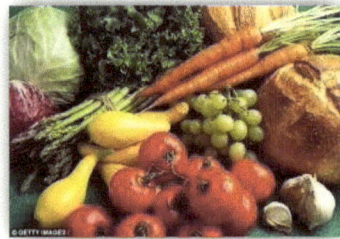

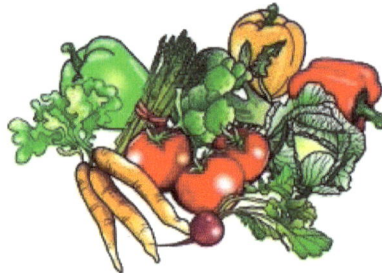

A Few Word Meanings

Radiesthesia: "the use of a divining rod in alternative medicine to identify appropriate herbal or homeopathic treatment"

Meninges:
"The three membranes (the dura mater, arachnoid, and pia mater) that line the skull and vertebral canal and enclose the brain and spinal cord."

Kelp:
"Kelps are large seaweeds belonging to the brown algae in the order Laminariales. There are about 30 different genera. Kelp grows in "underwater forests" in shallow oceans, and is thought to have appeared in the Miocene, 23 to 5 million years ago. The organisms require nutrient-rich water with temperatures between 6 and 14 °C. They are known for their high growth rate—the genera Macrocystis and Nereocystis can grow as fast as half a metre a day, ultimately reaching 30 to 80 metres."

Toxemia:
"Blood poisoning by toxins from a local bacterial infection."

Antispasmatic:
"This product contains several medications: belladonna alkaloids (made up of the drugs hyoscyamine, atropine, and scopolamine) and phenobarbital. Belladonna alkaloids help to reduce the symptoms of stomach and intestinal cramping. They work by slowing the natural movements of the gut and by relaxing the muscles in the stomach and intestines. Belladonna alkaloids belong to a class of drugs known as anticholinergics/antispasmodics. Phenobarbital helps to reduce anxiety. It acts on the brain to produce a calming effect. Phenobarbital belongs to a class of drugs known as barbiturate sedatives.
OTHER USES: This section contains uses of this drug that are not listed in the approved professional labeling for the drug but that may be prescribed by your health care professional. Use this drug for a condition that is listed in this section only if it has been so prescribed by your health care professional..."

Topics

Herbs to flush out body poisons.
Refresh & vitalize; Chilly and Sluggish; Weak hands; Restless legs
AMAZING BIBLE OIL CURE (FOR ARTHRITIS)
Energizing fragrances
Kelp the health Giver
Kelp as a Medicine
Kelp and the tissue salts
Kelp in nervous disorders
Kelp in headaches
Kelp in arterial troubles & high blood pressure
Indigestion and the pylorus
Kelp for weakness of the colon
Kelp vitalizes the important organs
Liver
Gall bladder & the pancreas
The bile duct & the kidneys
Prostate gland
The uterus
The testicles
The ovaries
Kelp and the thyroid
Kelp for Coughs, Colds, and Weak Lungs
The Best Way in which to Take Kelp and conclusion
Conclusion
Cinnamon and honey
ARTHRITIS, heart diseases, hair lose
BLADDER INFECTIONS, toothache
CHOLESTEROL, cold, indigestion
LONGEVITY, pimples, obesity, bad breath
Ginger Root and Honey health benefits
Some of the health benefits from Honey and Ginger Spice
Asthma Respiratory problems
Cancer Management, Cancer Prevention
Indigestion
Heart Health
Turmeric and its benefit
Turmeric Curcumin and what it is all about
Turmeric Curcumin possesses abilities
What we need in a Turmeric Curcumin Supplement
Powerful and Potency, Doctor Formulated
Maximum Absorption & No binder or fillers
Vegetable Capsules
Natural Ingredients
Things we should avoid when taking Turmeric. Also: Gelatin Capsule and fillers

Contents

IN CONCLUSION

Ms. Odessa has traveled the world; visiting many countries; she has even ventured the Mountains of Turkey.

"At my age I should have retired by now, but! I'm not; I have kept myself fit and healthy by using natural remedies and eating right; exercising and not allowing the stress of life to get me down; I love and enjoy helping people, and I relish the life God has given me. I have a BSN, MSN and an Honorary Masters and PHD. My prayer is that as you read everything in this health booklet that you will get the full benefit of it all."

Blessings to you,
From the desk of Ms. Odess

Ms. Odessa M. Frankson
RN/NURSE PRACTITIONER

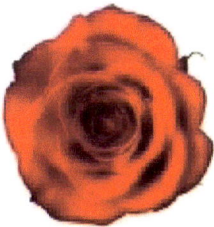

www.ingramcontent.com/pod-product-compliance
Lightning Source LLC
Chambersburg PA
CBHW060832270326
41933CB00002B/55